THE DOG GUARDIANS ESSENTIAL GUIDE TO USING BIOCHEMIC TISSUE SALTS

NATURAL HEALING FROM PUPPY TO SENIOR

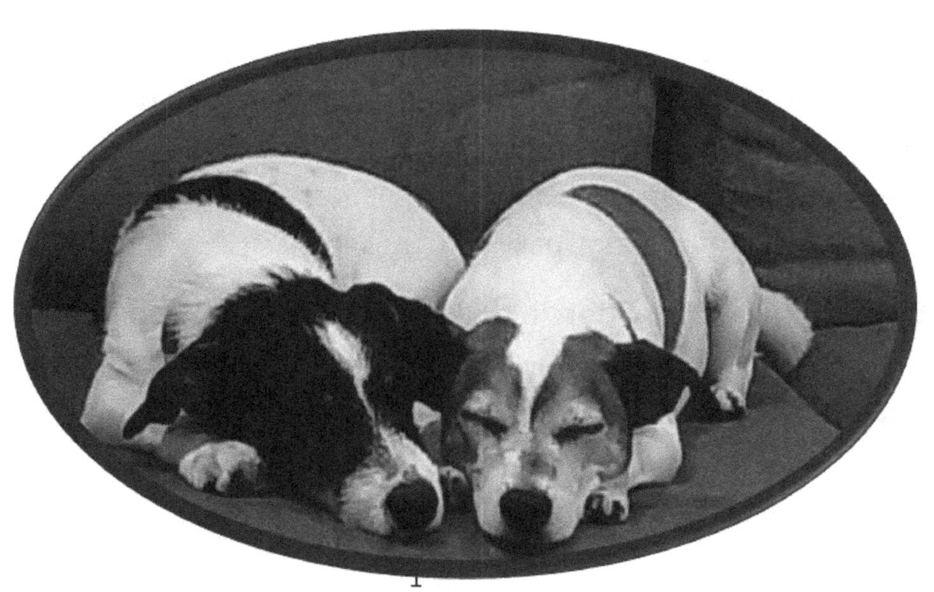

Disclaimer

This book is intended for educational and informational purposes only. The use of biochemic tissue salts as outlined in this guide is not intended to diagnose, treat, cure, or prevent any disease in animals. The content provided here does not replace professional veterinary advice, diagnosis, or treatment.

The information in this book is based on the author's personal experience and research, and it is recommended that pet owners consult with a licensed veterinarian for any specific concerns regarding their pet's health. The author is not a veterinarian, and this book does not serve as a substitute for veterinary care.

This guide is not intended to infringe upon any regulations set forth by the Veterinary Medicines Directorate (VMD) or the Royal College of Veterinary Surgeons (RCVS). It does not promote or encourage the unauthorized use of veterinary medicines or prescribe remedies outside the professional scope of qualified veterinary practitioners.

By using the information in this book, you acknowledge that the author is not liable for any outcomes or decisions made regarding the health of your pet.

About the author:

Shaz Ridler is an internationally published children's author, Homeopathic coach based in the West Country of the UK.

A dedicated animal lover, she is passionate about using homeopathy for both humans and animals, and empowering people to learn more so they can become a competent home user of all thing's homeopathy.

She has created a series of "How to" courses on her web site enabling complete novices to homeopathic remedies and their use become familiar with the simplified uses of homeopathic remedies.

The How to use the Homeopathic Pet Kit courses are popular as the course is broken down into easy-to-understand bite sized chunks to gradually build up your knowledge on the 24 homeopathic remedies contained with the Kit.

Over the years, shaz has shared her life with a wide variety of animals, from fish, rodents, rabbits and goats to horses and many species in between. Shaz has a particular fondness for dogs of all sizes, from the majestic St. Bernard to her small yet mighty Jack Russell terriers, and cannot imagine life without them. As a committed animal lover and homeopath, she provides educational guidance to pet guardians on the use of homeopathy to support their pets' overall wellbeing.

Discover a better way of healing paws and fur the homeopathic way.

Author contact www.Homeopathypetcoaching.com

Petcarecoach@gmail.com

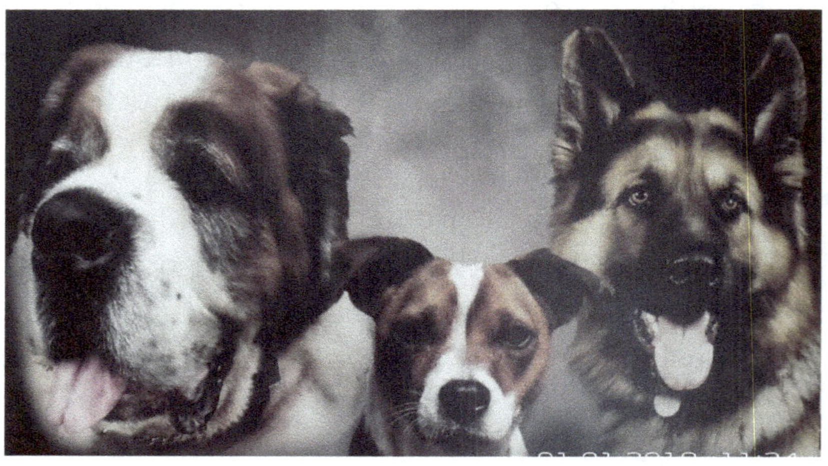

Acknowledgements

I would like to extend my heartfelt thanks to the late great Christopher Day, The best vet that ever walked this earth (imo) your work has truly motivated me to bring this project to life.

A special thanks to the amazing dogs with whom I have shared my life. You have taught me so much and continue to drive my passion for educating people to raise healthy animals.

To the readers and dog guardians, your dedication to the wellbeing of your furry friends is truly inspiring. This book is for you and your beloved dogs, and I hope it may help you provide the best support possible. Your commitment to natural and holistic health is what makes this journey worthwhile.

Contents

TISSUE SALTS FOR DOGS

Using tissue salts for dogs can form part of a holistic and gentle approach to support their health and well-being throughout various life stages. These essential minerals, known for their targeted cellular support, can address a range of common issues in dogs, including digestive sensitivities, joint health, anxiety, dental concerns, and more. From puppyhood to the senior years and even during the final stages of life, tissue salts offer a natural way to complement traditional veterinary care. By incorporating specific tissue salts into a dog's diet, pet guardians, breeders, and veterinarians can contribute to the overall vitality, comfort, and resilience of their canine companions, promoting a higher quality of life for these cherished members of the family.

Based on my experience as a homeopath and a devoted coach and guardian, I understand the significance of proactive healthcare for our canine companions. By integrating tissue salts and homeopathic remedies into my dogs' daily routines, I fortify their vital force, providing a preventative shield against common ailments that may surface over the course of their lives. This essential and easy-to-use guide is crafted to empower fellow dog guardians, enabling them to take a proactive stance in caring for their dogs, fostering the potential for long and vibrant lives in a simplistic way using the 12 biochemic Tissue Salts.

Tissue salts, also known as Biochemic cell salts or Schuessler salts

Tissue salts, also known as cell salts or Schuessler salts, are a unique class of therapeutic minerals that play a fundamental role in maintaining cellular health and balance within the body. The concept of tissue salts was developed by Dr. Wilhelm Heinrich Schuessler, a German physician, in the late 19th century.

Dr. Schuessler's groundbreaking work originated from the belief that imbalances in these vital minerals within the cells could lead to various health issues. His journey began with an observation of the cremated remains of human bodies, where he identified twelve essential minerals that were consistently present.

These minerals were then linked to specific biochemical functions in the body, forming the basis of Dr. Schuessler's theory of biochemistry and cell salts.

The twelve tissue salts identified by

Dr Schuessler are universally numbered as follows-
1. Calcium Fluoride
2. Calcium Phosphate
3. Calcium Sulphate
4. Ferrum Phosphate
5. Kali Muriaticum
6. Kali Phosphate
7. Kali Sulphate
8. Magnesia Phosphate
9. Natrum Muriaticum
10. Natrum Phosphate
11. Natrum Sulphate
12. Silicea

Dr. Schuessler's unique contribution was not just in identifying these minerals but in developing a method to make them bioavailable and easily assimilated by the cells. He prepared these minerals in a homeopathic form, reducing them to micro-doses for optimal absorption and utilisation at the cellular level. This process, known as potentisation, involves a series of dilutions and succussions, resulting in tissue salts that are gentle, safe, and effective.

Each tissue salt has specific functions and is associated with certain tissues or organs in the body. For example, Calcium Phosphate (Calc Phos) is linked to bone health, while Kali Phosphate (Kali Phos) is associated with nerve and brain function. Silicea is known for its role in maintaining skin, hair, and nail health. When the body is showing a deficiency of any of these salts within the body, they will show as particular issues. By looking at these Common issues and following this guide you can supplement the deficient tissue salt and regain balance.

These tissue salts are widely used to address a variety of health concerns in both humans and animals, including dogs. In dogs, tissue salts are often incorporated into their diets to support overall well-being, address specific health issues, and complement conventional veterinary care.

Tissue salts can be administered in various forms, such as tablets or powders, making them convenient for pet guardians to incorporate into a dog's daily routine. The versatility and broad range of applications make tissue salts a popular choice for those seeking a natural and holistic approach to health and wellness for their canine companions. They can be given by tipping a pill into the side of the jowls and most dogs will happily take them from the floor. Crushing them between 2 spoons will also work as well and then administering as a powder to the dog.

Tissue salts, founded by Dr. Wilhelm Heinrich Schuessler, represent a holistic and biochemic approach to cellular health. Their origin lies in meticulous observations and a profound understanding of the crucial role these minerals play in maintaining balance within the body. Today, tissue salts are recognised for their versatility and efficacy in supporting health across various species, offering a natural complement to conventional veterinary care.

Tissue salts are usually in a 6X potency and can be purchased from some health food shops, online and homeopathic pharmacies. Helios Homeopathic pharmacy have created their own range of tissue salts.

Elevating Canine Wellness

The Impact of Tissue Salts for Working Dogs, Breeding Canines, and Cherished Companions

In the Canine world of health, a proactive and holistic approach is paramount. As the roles of working dogs, breeding canines, and cherished companions continue to evolve, many pet guardians are turning to holistic solutions. Tissue salts, known for their targeted cellular support, are gaining popularity for promoting the well-being of dogs. This book explores the versatile applications of tissue salts across different canine categories—working dogs, breeding canines, and pets—illustrating their potential to elevate canine health.

Understanding Tissue Salts

Tissue salts, or Schüssler salts, consist of 12 essential minerals crucial for cellular function. These minerals, when utilised in homeopathic dilutions, address imbalances at the cellular level, promoting overall health and well-being. Let's delve into how tissue salts can be beneficial for canine health in various contexts.

Potency and where to purchase

Tissue salts are usually in a 6X or 12X potency and can be purchased from some health food shops, online and homeopathic pharmacies. Some Homeopathic pharmacies' have created their own range of tissue salts.

Important Notes Before Starting Tissue Salts for Your Pet

Nature of the Health Issue: If your pet has a chronic condition, is on prescribed medication, or has multiple health concerns requiring medical supervision, consult their vet before using cell salts.

Type of Health Issue: Cell salts are generally safe for skin, fur, digestion, and musculoskeletal support in pets. Consult with your vet for further advice.

Avoid These Forms: Do not use liquid cell salts containing ethanol or alcohol, as these are toxic to cats and dogs. For pets with food allergies, avoid lactose-based tablets to prevent allergic reactions.

Best Ways to Administer Cell Salts to your Pet.

For cooperative pets, crush a few pellets between two spoons and place the powder directly in their mouth (dry dose).

Some dogs may let you place the pellets between their front teeth and lower lip to dissolve.

For less tolerant pets, dissolve crushed pellets in a small amount of water and use a plastic syringe to administer it.

Alternatively, you can add 3-5 crushed doses to their water bowl, stirring well (plussing method).

Dosage Guidelines:

Give 1-3 doses daily. For acute complaints, administer every 30 minutes to 2 hours, up to 12 doses in a day, for no more than a couple of days. If needed longer, consult your vet.

How to Know If Cell Salts Are Working
As a general rule: 6 doses for recent issues or 6 weeks for chronic conditions. If improvement isn't noticeable, stop.

For chronic issues, follow a dosing cycle: 5 days on, 2 days off.

When to Stop:
Once you see improvement, gradually reduce the dosage and stop when it's no longer needed. Unlike traditional medications, homeopathic remedies should be tapered off as issues resolve.

Repetition
The normal dosage is one pill three to four times per day. Place the pill directly into the mouth and allow them to dissolve. These can be taken for 2 to 6 months for long standing complaints.
For the more acute issues which arise then the dosses can be repeated every 30

minutes or so until improvement is seen. If there is no improvement after 4 to 6 doses then stop and look at the issues again and maybe choose another tissue salt.

Decide the tissue salt on the issues which are standing out. These can be continued for 2 to 7 days.

Disclaimer
This book is designed to complement the care provided by your veterinarian for your dog. Collaborating with a homeopathic or holistic vet can greatly benefit your pet, and their advice should always be sought for guidance and treatment. The purpose of this book is to educate you about tissue salts and their applications, and it is not a replacement for professional veterinary care.

Working Dogs: Maximising Performance and Wellbeing

Joint and Muscle Support: Magnesia Phosphorica (Mag Phos) aids in preventing muscle cramps and spasms, supporting the joint and muscle health necessary for the physical demands placed on working dogs.

Digestive Resilience: Natrum phosphoricum (Nat Phos) regulates pH balance, aiding in preventing acidosis and supporting healthy digestion during strenuous work.

Breeding Canines:
Fostering Reproductive Vitality:
-Reproductive Health: Silicea supports reproductive organ health, aiding in preventing infections and maintaining overall reproductive well-being in breeding canines.

Stress Management: Kali phosphoricum (Kali Phos) alleviates stress, creating an environment conducive to optimal breeding conditions.

Pets: Wellness for Beloved Companions

Joint and Bone Health: Calcarea Phosphorica (Calc Phos) supports bone development, ensuring structural integrity for the overall health and comfort of pets.

Digestive Harmony: Natrum phosphoricum (Nat Phos) regulates pH balance, aiding in preventing acidosis and supporting healthy digestion in pets.

Immune Resilience: Ferrum phosphoricum (Ferr Phos) enhances oxygenation, fortifying the immune system for overall health resilience in pets.

Incorporating Tissue Salts into Canine Health Management:

Whether managing a team of working dogs, a breeding program, or a cherished pet, integrating tissue salts into the health management plan involves thoughtful consideration. Pet guardians can collaborate with veterinarians to devise a targeted supplementation plan based on the specific needs and challenges faced by their canine companions. Regular monitoring and adjustments ensure ongoing support tailored to individual health requirements.

Navigating the complexities of canine health requires a holistic and forward-thinking approach. Tissue salts, with their targeted cellular support, offer a promising avenue for enhancing the well-being of working dogs, breeding canines, and pets alike. By addressing specific health concerns and promoting overall vitality, tissue salts contribute to the holistic health and happiness of our canine companions, ushering in a new era of well-being in the diverse world of canine care.

Optimising Canine Health: Unveiling the Potential of the 12 Main Tissue Salts for Dogs

In the pursuit of a more natural and holistic canine care, many pet guardians are exploring alternative avenues to support their furry companions' well-being. Among these, the use of tissue salts and Homeopathy is gaining attention with several dedicated online groups to help guardians learn of a more natural approach to pet husbandry.

These 12 essential minerals offer targeted cellular support, addressing imbalances at a fundamental level. In this book we delve into how the main 12 tissue salts can benefit dogs, promoting overall health and vitality.

Let's take a closer look at their individual Tissue salts and some of their indications.

1. **Calcarea Fluorica (Calc. Fluor.)**

Key Uses: Strengthening bones, teeth, and connective tissues.

Joint and Bone Issues: Calc. Fluor. is beneficial for dogs with weak or deformed bones, bone spurs, and arthritis. It may help in strengthening the skeletal structure, making it useful for growing puppies and older dogs with arthritis. Supports the strength and flexibility of joints and ligaments, crucial for dogs, especially active breeds prone to musculoskeletal issues.
Dental Health: It aids in the maintenance of strong teeth and can be helpful in cases of dental decay or weak teeth in dogs.
Ligament and Tendon Health: Supports the elasticity of ligaments and tendons, aiding in conditions like hip dysplasia and other joint disorders.
Health Conditions Supported:
Hip dysplasia in puppies and adult dogs.
Arthritis and joint pain in senior dogs.
Dental issues like weak or decaying teeth.
Ligament injuries and sprains.

2. Calcarea Phosphorica (Calc. Phos.)

Key Uses: Bone growth, teething, and general development.

Growth Support: Essential for puppies during growth spurts to ensure proper bone development.
Teething: Relieves discomfort associated with teething in puppies and may help with the formation of strong teeth. - Healing: Aids in the healing of fractures and other bone injuries.

Health Conditions Supported:
Growth pains in puppies.
Teething discomfort.
Delayed bone healing after fractures.
Weak bones in aging dogs.
Digestive disorders due to poor assimilation.

3. Calcarea Sulph (Calc. Sulph.)

Key Uses: Skin and wound healing.

Skin Conditions: May help skin infections, abscesses, and wounds that are slow to heal.

Wound Healing: Aids in wound healing and skin conditions, providing support for dogs recovering from injuries or dealing with skin irritations.

Pus Formation: May help in conditions where there is a discharge of pus, indicating its use in helping abscesses and boils.

Health Conditions Supported:
Skin infections like pyoderma.
Abscesses and boils.
Slow-healing wounds.
Chronic ear infections with pus.
Skin and ear abscess.
Suppurating wounds.
Conjunctivitis with thick yellow discharge.

4. Ferrum Phosphoricum (Ferr. Phos.)
Key Uses: Inflammation, fever, and infections.

Early Stages of Inflammation: Useful in the initial stages of any inflammatory condition.
Fever: Reduces fever and may help in managing infections. - Respiratory Issues: Assists in helping respiratory infections and conditions like bronchitis.
Enhanced Oxygenation: Improves oxygenation in the blood, supporting the immune system and overall vitality, especially beneficial for energetic and working dogs.

Health Conditions Supported:
Early stages of colds and infections.
Fever management.
Bronchitis and respiratory infections.
General inflammation.
Mastitis.
Inflamed larynx or trachea.

5. Kali Muriaticum (Kali Mur.)

Key Uses: Congestion, glandular swelling, and digestive issues.

Respiratory Congestion: May help in cases of nasal congestion and catarrh.
Glandular Swelling: Reduces swelling of glands, making it useful for conditions like swollen lymph nodes. - Digestive Issues: Aids in digestive disorders such as constipation and indigestion.
Immune Support: Boosts the immune system, aiding in resistance against common infections, making it beneficial for dogs prone to respiratory or skin issues.

Health Conditions Supported:
Nasal congestion and sinusitis.
Swollen lymph nodes.
Indigestion and constipation.
Ear infections with white discharge.
Indigestion after eating fatty foods.
Vaccination adverse reactions.

6. Kali Phosphoricum (Kali Phos.)

Key Uses: Nervous system support, mental health, and fatigue.

Nervous Conditions: May help in managing nervous disorders, anxiety, and depression in dogs.
Fatigue: Alleviates issues of fatigue and exhaustion.
Mental Alertness: Promotes mental clarity and alertness.
Stress Reduction: Alleviates stress and nervousness, promoting a calm and balanced demeanour, essential for dogs facing anxiety or environmental stressors.

Health Conditions Supported

Anxiety and nervousness in dogs.
Fatigue and general weakness.
Behavioural issues stemming from nervous disorders.
Depression and lack of vitality.
Involuntary urination.
Nerve degeneration.

7. Kali Sulphuricum (Kali Sulph.)
 Key Uses: Skin conditions, respiratory issues, and detoxification.

Skin Disorders: May help skin diseases characterised by scaling and desquamation.
Respiratory Problems: Aids in the relief of chronic respiratory issues.
Cellular Detoxification: Supports cellular detoxification and contributes to skin health, making it useful for dogs with skin conditions.
Supports the body's detoxification processes.

Health Conditions Supported:
Chronic skin conditions like eczema and dermatitis.
Asthma and chronic bronchitis.
Detoxification support in dogs exposed to toxins.
Dandruff and scaly skin.
Urticaria rash – Nettle rash.

8. Magnesia Phosphorica (Mag. Phos.)
Key Uses: Muscle cramps, spasms, and pain relief.

Muscle Cramps: Relieves muscle cramps and spasms.
Muscle Health: Aids in preventing muscle cramps and spasms, supporting overall muscle health, especially beneficial for active and working dogs.
Pain Relief: Alleviates pain from various sources, including digestive colic and menstrual cramps.
Nerve Pain: May help in managing nerve-related pain.

Health Conditions Supported:
Muscle cramps and spasms.
Digestive colic and abdominal pain.
Nerve pain and neuralgia.
Restless leg syndrome in dogs.
Colic.

9. Natrum Muriaticum (Nat. Mur.)
Key Uses: Fluid balance, digestive health, and skin conditions.

Fluid Retention: May help in conditions of water retention and dehydration.
Digestive Health: Supports proper digestion and alleviates constipation.
Skin Health: May help dry and flaky skin conditions.
Electrolyte Balance: Regulates electrolyte balance, crucial for hydration and preventing issues related to dehydration, particularly important for active dogs.

Health Conditions Supported:
Dehydration and fluid imbalance.
Constipation and digestive disorders.
Dry skin and eczema.
Allergies and hay fever.
Dry Nose
Oedema
Seaside asthma

10. Natrum Phosphoricum (Nat. Phos.)
Key Uses: Acid-base balance, digestive issues, and joint health.

Acid Neutralisation: May help in neutralising excess stomach acid, aiding in digestive disorders.
Acid-Base Balance: Regulates pH balance, aiding in digestion and preventing acidosis, beneficial for dogs with digestive sensitivities or prone to stomach upset.
Joint Health: Supports the health of joints and alleviates issues of arthritis.
Urinary Health: Prevents the formation of urate crystals and stones in the urinary tract.

Health Conditions Supported:
Acid reflux and heartburn.
Arthritis and joint pain.
Urinary tract infections and stones.
Gout and related conditions.
Milk Allergy

11. Natrum Sulphuricum (Nat. Sulph.)

Key Uses: Liver health, detoxification, and respiratory issues.

Liver Support: Supports liver function and detoxification, contributing to overall metabolic health, particularly important for dogs with liver concerns.
Respiratory Health: May help respiratory conditions like asthma and bronchitis.
Digestive Aid: Supports the digestive system and alleviates issues with indigestion.

Health Conditions Supported:
Liver diseases and jaundice.
Asthma and chronic respiratory conditions.
Indigestion and bloating.
Toxin exposure and detoxification.
Oedema of the lower legs and feet.
Water retention

12. Silicea (Silica)

Key Uses: Skin and connective tissue health, immune support, and expulsion of foreign bodies.

Immune Support: Enhances the immune system's ability to fight infections.
Expulsion of Foreign Bodies: May help in the expulsion of splinters and other foreign objects from the body.
Connective Tissue Health: Promotes the health of connective tissues and aids in preventing infections, beneficial for dogs with skin issues or those recovering from injuries.

Health Conditions Supported:
Chronic skin conditions like eczema and abscesses.
Weak immune system and recurrent infections.
Splinters and embedded foreign bodies.
Fistulas and chronic discharges.
Seborrhoea – oily skin.

Dosage and Administration

Potency: Biochemic tissue salts are typically administered in low potencies, such as 6X or 12X.

Frequency: For acute conditions, the popular guidelines are that tissue salts can be given every ½ hour or 1-2 hours until improvement is seen.
For chronic conditions, they can be administered 2-3 times daily.
Day 1-5: Take 1-3 times per day.
Day 6-7: Rest days (no cell salts).
Example Take 1 cell salt three times per day on Monday to Friday, take rest days on the weekend. Repeat as necessary.

When to Stop Taking Cell Salts
As issues improve, reduce the frequency of cell salts. Once fully resolved, discontinue use

Administration: The salts can be dissolved in water and given directly into the dog's mouth or mixed with their food.

Specific Support and Dosages

Joint and Bone Health:
Calc. Fluor. 6X: Twice daily for joint pain and bone issues.   - Calc. Phos. 6X: Twice daily for growing puppies or dogs recovering from fractures.

Skin Conditions:
Calc. Sulph. 6X: Three times daily for abscesses and slow healing wounds.
Kali Sulph. 6X: Twice daily for chronic skin conditions like eczema.

Digestive Issues:
Kali Mur. 6X: Twice daily for constipation and digestive upsets.
Nat. Phos. 6X: Three times daily for acid reflux and digestive discomfort.

Respiratory Health:
Ferr. Phos. 6X: Every 1-2 hours during acute respiratory infections.

Nat. Sulph. 6X: Twice daily for chronic respiratory conditions like asthma.

Nervous System Support:
Kali Phos. 6X: Twice daily for anxiety and nervousness.

Incorporating Tissue Salts into Canine Care

Pet guardians interested in integrating tissue salts into their dog's care regimen should consult with veterinarians to develop a tailored supplementation plan. Regular observation of the dog's health and behaviour allows for adjustments to the plan, ensuring a holistic and personalised approach to canine well-being.

The main 12 tissue salts present a holistic approach to canine care, addressing various aspects of a dog's health from bone strength to immune support. By understanding the specific benefits each salt offers, pet guardians can optimise their dog's health, promoting a vibrant and happy life for their cherished companions.

Harmonising the Canine Reproductive Cycle

Tissue Salts for Supporting a Bitch's Season

The reproductive health of female dogs, especially during their breeding seasons, is a critical aspect of responsible canine care. In this exploration of tissue salts' potential, we delve into how these essential minerals can play a supportive role in addressing ailments and issues associated with a bitch's reproductive cycle. From mood swings to physical discomfort, tissue salts offer a holistic approach to nurturing the well-being of our canine companions.

Understanding the Canine Reproductive Cycle

A bitch's reproductive cycle is marked by distinct phases, including proestrus, oestrus, dioestrus, and anoestrus. Each stage involves hormonal fluctuations and physiological changes that can impact the dog's behaviour and overall health. Tissue salts can offer targeted support during these phases.

Common Ailments and Issues

Mood Swings and Stress:

Common issues may include: Behavioural changes, restlessness, and increased stress.

Tissue Salt: Kali phosphoricum (Kali Phos) May help alleviate stress and nervousness, promoting a more balanced and relaxed demeanour during the reproductive cycle.

Digestive Upsets:

Issues: Digestive issues, including bloating or changes in appetite.

Tissue Salt: Natrum phosphoricum (Nat Phos) regulates pH balance, aiding in digestion and preventing acidosis, which can contribute to digestive discomfort.

Muscular Cramps and Discomfort:

Common issues may include: Physical discomfort, muscular cramps, or spasms. Reluctance to walk or jump and not being able to get comfortable.

Tissue Salt: Magnesia Phosphorica (Mag Phos) aids in preventing muscle cramps and spasms, providing relief from physical discomfort.

Hormonal Imbalance:
Common may include: Irregularities in the reproductive cycle or hormonal imbalances. Loss of appetite and hiding away.

Tissue Salt: Silicea supports hormonal balance, contributing to a more regulated and harmonious reproductive system.

Immune System Support:
Common issues may include: Increased vulnerability to infections during the reproductive cycle.

Tissue Salt: Ferrum phosphoricum (Ferr Phos) enhances oxygenation, supporting a robust immune response to prevent and combat infections.

Incorporating Tissue Salts into Canine Care during the reproductive Cycle:

Pet guardians, breeders, and veterinarians can collaborate to develop a targeted supplementation plan using tissue salts during a bitch's reproductive cycle. Observing the dog's behaviour and physical well-being closely allows for adjustments to the supplementation plan as needed.

Tissue salts provide a holistic and natural approach to supporting a bitch's reproductive health, addressing a range of issues and discomfort associated with the various phases of the reproductive cycle. By incorporating these essential minerals into the care routine, pet guardians can contribute to the overall well-being and comfort of their canine companions during this crucial aspect of their lives.

Navigating Canine Mating with Ease

Tissue Salts for Supporting Bitches

The process of mating in dogs is a crucial phase in their reproductive journey, and ensuring the well-being of the bitch during this time is paramount. Tissue salts, with their targeted cellular support, emerge as valuable allies in addressing potential problems, ailments, and issue's associated with mating. This section delves into how tissue salts can play a supportive role in facilitating a smoother and more comfortable mating experience for bitches.

Understanding Canine Mating Challenges:

The mating process in dogs can present various challenges for bitches, ranging from physical discomfort to stress-related issue's. Tissue salts offer a natural and holistic approach to addressing these challenges.

Common Ailments and Issue's During Mating

Stress and Anxiety:
Common issue's may include: Behavioural changes, restlessness, and increased stress.

Tissue Salt: Kali phosphoricum (Kali Phos) may help alleviate stress and nervousness, promoting a calm and relaxed demeanour during the mating process.

Digestive Discomfort:
Common issues may include: Digestive issues such as indigestion or changes in appetite.

Tissue Salt: Natrum phosphoricum (Nat Phos) regulates pH balance, aiding in digestion and preventing acidosis, which can contribute to digestive discomfort during mating.

Muscular Cramps and Strain:
Physical discomfort, muscular cramps, or strain.

Tissue Salt Magnesia Phosphorica (Mag Phos) aids in preventing muscle cramps and spasms, providing relief from physical discomfort associated with mating.

Hormonal Imbalances:
Irregularities in hormonal balance during mating.

Tissue Salt: Silicea supports hormonal balance, contributing to a more regulated and harmonious reproductive system.

Immune Support:
 Increased vulnerability to infections during mating.

Tissue Salt: Ferrum phosphoricum (Ferr Phos) enhances oxygenation, supporting a robust immune response to prevent and combat infections that may occur during the mating process.

Incorporating Tissue Salts into Canine Mating Care:

Pet guardians, breeders, and veterinarians can collaborate to design a targeted supplementation plan using tissue salts during the mating phase. Close observation of the bitch's behaviour and physical condition allows for adjustments to the supplementation plan as needed.

Tissue salts provide a gentle and natural approach to supporting bitches during the mating process, addressing a range of potential challenges and discomforts. By incorporating these essential minerals into the care routine, pet guardians can contribute to the overall well-being and comfort of their canine companions during this crucial aspect of their reproductive journey and ensuring that she is in optimum health before the mating process begins.

Nurturing Canine Maternity

Tissue Salts as Guardians through the Stages of Pregnancy

Pregnancy in dogs is a transformative and delicate period that demands careful attention to the well-being of the expecting bitch. Tissue salts, renowned for their targeted cellular support, emerge as essential allies in safeguarding the health of the pregnant dog. This section explores how tissue salts can play a crucial role in supporting bitches through the various stages of pregnancy, addressing potential problems, ailments, and issue's to ensure a smooth and comfortable journey to motherhood.

Understanding Canine Pregnancy Challenges:

Each stage of pregnancy in dogs comes with its unique set of challenges, from hormonal fluctuations to physical strain.

Tissue salts offer a natural and holistic approach to alleviating these challenges. A typical gestation period for a bitch from mating to whelping (giving birth) is 63 days (9 weeks) There are several online dog pregnancy calculators which may help determine a due date for whelping.

Common Ailments and suport During Canine Pregnancy:
Nausea and Digestive Discomfort:
Issue's: Morning sickness, nausea, and potential digestive upset.

Tissue Salt: Natrum phosphoricum (Nat Phos) regulates pH balance, aiding in digestion and preventing acidosis, offering relief from nausea and digestive discomfort.

Muscular Strain and Fatigue:
Issue's: Physical discomfort, muscular strain, and fatigue.

Tissue Salt: Magnesia Phosphorica (Mag Phos) aids in preventing muscle cramps and spasms, providing relief from muscular discomfort and fatigue during pregnancy.

Stress and Anxiety:
Behavioural changes, restlessness, and increased stress.

Tissue Salt: Kali phosphoricum (Kali Phos) may help alleviate stress and nervousness, promoting a calm and relaxed demeanour for the pregnant bitch.

Hormonal Imbalances:
Irregularities in hormonal balance during pregnancy.

Tissue Salt: Silicea supports hormonal balance, contributing to a more regulated and harmonious reproductive system.

Immune Support:
Increased vulnerability to infections during pregnancy.

Tissue Salt: Ferrum phosphoricum (Ferr Phos) enhances oxygenation, supporting a robust immune response to prevent and combat infections that may occur during pregnancy.

Supporting the Miracle of Birth

Support Through Canine Whelping

The whelping process is a defining moment in a canine's life, demanding careful attention and support for both the mother and her newborns. Tissue salts, recognised for their targeted cellular support, stand as invaluable aids during the stages of whelping. In this section, we explore how tissue salts can play a pivotal role in supporting bitches through the whelping process, addressing potential problems, and issues to ensure a safe and comfortable birthing experience.

Understanding Canine Whelping Challenges:

Whelping involves a series of intricate stages, each presenting unique challenges for the mother. From labour pains to postpartum recovery, tissue salts offer a holistic approach to easing the physical and emotional strains associated with whelping.

Common Issue's During Canine Whelping

Labor Pains and Muscular Discomfort:

Intense labour pains, muscular strain, and discomfort.

Tissue Salt: Magnesia Phosphorica (Mag Phos) aids in preventing muscle cramps and spasms, providing relief from labour-related muscular discomfort.

Fatigue and Energy Depletion:

Exhaustion and energy depletion during the birthing process.

Tissue Salt: Ferrum phosphoricum (Ferr Phos) enhances oxygenation, supporting energy levels and vitality during whelping.

Stress and Anxiety:

Common Issue's may include: Increased stress and anxiety during labour and delivery.

Tissue Salt: Kali phosphoricum (Kali Phos) may help alleviate stress and nervousness, promoting a calm and focused demeanour for the mother.

Hormonal Imbalances:
Fluctuations in hormonal balance during and after whelping.

Tissue Salt: Silicea supports hormonal balance, aiding in a smooth transition through the hormonal shifts associated with whelping.

Immune Support:
Vulnerability to infections postpartum.

Tissue Salt: Natrum phosphoricum (Nat Phos) regulates pH balance, supporting the immune system and preventing infections during the recovery period.

Incorporating Tissue Salts into Canine Whelping Care:
Tissue salts serve as reliable allies in supporting bitches through the multifaceted challenges of whelping.

By addressing potential problems and providing natural relief from discomfort, tissue salts contribute to a smoother, safer, and more comfortable birthing experience for both the mother and her newborns. In embracing these essential minerals, pet guardians can ensure the

well-being of their canine companions
during this profound and miraculous
event.

Nurturing the Next Generation

Tissue salts Guardians Through a Puppy's First Weeks of Life

The first few weeks of a puppy's life mark a critical period of growth and development, requiring meticulous care to ensure their health and vitality. Tissue salts, renowned for their targeted cellular support, emerge as crucial companions in addressing potential problems, and issues during this delicate phase. This section explores how tissue salts can play an integral role in supporting puppies through their initial weeks of life, including addressing the concerning issue of failure to thrive.

Understanding Puppy Development Challenges:

From birth to weaning, a puppy undergoes rapid physical and behavioural changes. Tissue salts offer a holistic approach to addressing potential challenges and ensuring the well-being of the young canine.

Common support During a Puppy's First Weeks:
Failure to Thrive:
Common Issue's may include: Insufficient weight gain, lethargy, and a lack of developmental progress.

Tissue Salt: Calcarea Phosphorica (Calc Phos) supports bone and overall development, aiding in overcoming the challenges associated with failure to thrive in puppies.
Digestive Sensitivities:
Issue's: Upset stomach, diarrhoea, or constipation.

Tissue Salt: Natrum phosphoricum (Nat Phos) regulates pH balance, aiding in digestion and preventing acidosis, providing relief from digestive discomfort.

Muscular Cramps and Discomfort:
Issue's: Restlessness, discomfort, or signs of muscle tension.

Tissue Salt: Magnesia Phosphorica (Mag Phos) aids in preventing muscle cramps and spasms, promoting comfort and relaxation for the growing puppy.

Immune Vulnerability:
Increased susceptibility to infections.

Tissue Salt: Ferrum phosphoricum (Ferr Phos) enhances oxygenation, supporting a robust immune response and preventing infections in the early weeks of a puppy's life.

Teething Discomfort:
Common Issues may include: Chewing, drooling, and signs of teething discomfort. Reluctance to eat.

Tissue Salt: Calcarea Fluorica (Calc Fluor) supports dental health and may provide relief during the teething phase.

Incorporating Tissue Salts into Puppy Care:

Tissue salts serve as gentle and natural allies in supporting puppies during the puppy's first weeks of life. Regular observation of the puppy's behaviour and physical condition allows for adjustments to the supplementation plan as needed. By incorporating these essential minerals into the care routine, pet guardians can recognise the potential challenges and promote the overall well-being as well as contribute to the healthy development and resilience of their young canine companions, ensuring a strong and vibrant start to life.

Building Resilience in Puppies:

Tissue Salts as Guardians from 3 to 8 Weeks of Life

The period from 3 to 8 weeks of a puppy's life is a crucial stage marked by significant developmental milestones, including weaning and the introduction of vaccinations if being used. Tissue salts, play a vital role in fostering resilience during this transitional phase. This section explores how tissue salts can address potential problems, and issues, including the ongoing concerning issue of failure to thrive and supporting a puppy's response to vaccinations.

Understanding the Challenges of Weeks 3 to 8:

As puppies transition from dependence on their mother's milk to solid food and receive essential vaccinations, various challenges may arise. Tissue salts offer a natural and holistic approach to addressing these challenges.

Common support needed in Puppies from 3 to 8 Weeks:

Failure to Thrive:

Common issues may include: Lack of weight gain, reduced energy, and slow development.

Tissue Salt: Calcarea Phosphorica (Calc Phos) supports bone development and overall growth, aiding in overcoming the challenges associated with failure to thrive in puppies.

Digestive Sensitivities:

Common Issue's may include: Upset stomach, diarrhoea, or constipation during the transition to solid food.

Tissue Salt: Natrum phosphoricum (Nat Phos) regulates pH balance, aiding in digestion and preventing acidosis, providing relief from digestive discomfort.

Teething Discomfort:

Some main Issue's include: Chewing, drooling, and signs of teething discomfort.

Tissue Salt: Calcarea Fluorica (Calc Fluor) supports dental health and may provide relief during the teething phase.

Vaccination Response:
Common Issue's may include: Mild discomfort, lethargy, or temporary changes in behaviour post-vaccination.

Any adverse reactions should be reported to your vet.

Tissue Salt: Ferrum phosphoricum (Ferr Phos) enhances oxygenation, supporting a balanced immune response and helping to alleviate mild post-vaccination issue's.

Stress and Anxiety:
Behavioural changes, restlessness, and increased stress during new experiences.

Tissue Salt: Kali phosphoricum (Kali Phos) may help alleviate stress and nervousness, promoting a calm and balanced demeanour during new and potentially stressful situations.

Incorporating Tissue Salts into Puppy Care:
Pet guardians, breeders, and veterinarians can collaborate to design a targeted supplementation plan using tissue salts during the critical weeks from 3 to 8. Regular observation of the puppy's

behaviour and physical condition allows
for adjustments to the supplementation
plan as needed.

Tissue salts serve as invaluable allies in supporting
puppies through the dynamic phase from 3 to 8 weeks,
addressing potential challenges associated with
growth, digestion, teething, and vaccinations. By
incorporating these essential minerals into the care
routine, pet guardians can contribute to the overall
well-being, resilience, and adaptability of their young
canine companions during this crucial stage of
development.

Thriving Through the Puppy Journey

Tissue Salts as Pillars of Support from 8 Weeks to the First Year

The journey from 8 weeks to the first year of a puppy's life is a dynamic and transformative period filled with numerous milestones and adjustments. Tissue salts, become indispensable allies in fostering the well-being, resilience, and adaptability of puppies during this crucial phase. This section explores how tissue salts can address potential problems, and issue's across various aspects, including vaccination and microchipping responses, teething, dietary changes, the transition from the litter and mother, anxiety, settling into a new home, and the early stages of puppy training.

Understanding the Challenges of Puppyhood (8 Weeks to 1 Year):
This developmental stage involves a series of changes, both physical and psychological, as puppies adapt to new environments, experiences, and routines. It is a pivotal time in a young pup's life and one stage which should be handled with care.

Common support issues in Puppies from 8 Weeks to 1 Year:
Vaccination and Microchipping Responses:
Mild discomfort, lethargy, or behavioural changes post-vaccination and microchipping.

Tissue Salt: Ferrum phosphoricum (Ferr Phos) enhances oxygenation, supporting a balanced immune response and aiding in the alleviation of mild post-vaccination issue's.

Teething Discomfort:
Chewing, drooling, and signs of teething discomfort.

Tissue Salt: Calcarea Fluorica (Calc Fluor) supports dental health and may provide relief during the teething phase.

Food Changes:
Digestive upset during transitions to new diets.

Tissue Salt: Natrum phosphoricum (Nat Phos) regulates pH balance, aiding in digestion and preventing acidosis, providing relief from digestive discomfort during food changes.

Leaving Litter and Mother:
Common Issue's may include Anxiety, restlessness, and difficulty adjusting to a new environment.

Tissue Salt: Kali phosphoricum (Kali Phos) may help alleviate stress and nervousness, promoting a calm demeanour during the transition to a new home.

Settling into a New Home:
Behavioural challenges, anxiety, and difficulty adapting to a new environment.

Tissue Salt: Kali muriaticum (Kali Mur) aids in adapting to new surroundings, supporting emotional balance during the settling-in period.

Puppy Training:
Behavioural challenges, resistance to training, or difficulty focusing.

Tissue Salt: Kali phosphoricum (Kali Phos) can enhance mental alertness and focus, facilitating the learning process during puppy training.

Incorporating Tissue Salts into Puppy Care:
Pet guardians, breeders, and veterinarians can collaborate to design a targeted supplementation plan using tissue salts throughout a puppy's first year. Regular observation of the puppy's behaviour and physical condition allows for adjustments to the supplementation plan as needed.

By providing targeted support for immune health, teething, dietary transitions, and emotional well-being, tissue salts will contribute to the overall health and adaptability of young canine companions.

Navigating Adolescence

Tissue Salts in the Journey from 1 Year to Adulthood

The transition from puppyhood to adolescence is a pivotal period in a dog's life, marked by physical growth, behavioural changes, and new experiences. Tissue salts, become essential companions during this developmental stage. This section explores how tissue salts can address a range of challenges, dietary transitions, puppy training, destructive behaviours like chewing furniture, fears such as fireworks, travel sickness, and anticipatory anxiety about veterinary visits, car rides, or holidays.

Understanding the Challenges of Adolescence:
Adolescent dogs experience a variety of challenges as they continue to grow physically and emotionally. Tissue salts offer a natural and holistic approach to support their overall wellbeing.

Common support issues in Dogs from 1 Year to Adolescence:
Vaccination boosters
Mild discomfort, lethargy, or behavioural changes post-vaccination.

Tissue Salt: Ferrum phosphoricum (Ferr Phos) enhances oxygenation, supporting a balanced immune response and aiding in the alleviation of mild post-vaccination issue's.

Food Changes:
Issue's: Digestive upset during transitions to new diets.

Tissue Salt: Natrum phosphoricum (Nat Phos) regulates pH balance, aiding in digestion and preventing acidosis, providing relief from digestive discomfort during food changes.

Puppy Training:
Behavioural challenges, resistance to training, or difficulty focusing.

Tissue Salt: Kali phosphoricum (Kali Phos) can enhance mental alertness and focus, facilitating the learning process during training sessions.

Chewing Furniture:

Issues: Destructive chewing behaviours.

Tissue Salt: Calcarea Fluorica (Calc Fluor) supports dental health and may provide relief during teething, potentially reducing the inclination to chew on furniture.

Firework Fears:

Common Issue's may include: Anxiety, restlessness, or fear during fireworks.

Tissue Salt: Kali phosphoricum (Kali Phos) may help alleviate stress and nervousness, promoting a calm demeanour during anxiety-inducing events like fireworks.

Travel Sickness:

Nausea, vomiting, drooling or discomfort during car rides.

Tissue Salt: Natrum phosphoricum (Nat Phos) regulates pH balance, aiding in digestion and preventing acidosis, providing relief from travel sickness.

Anticipatory Anxiety:
Common Issue's may include Stress,
restlessness, or fear associated with
upcoming events like vet visits or travel.

Tissue Salt: Kali phosphoricum (Kali Phos)
may help alleviate anticipatory anxiety,
promoting a more balanced and calm
state of mind.

Incorporating Tissue Salts into Adolescent Dog Care:
Pet guardians, trainers, and veterinarians
can collaborate and plan using tissue salts
during the adolescent stage. Regular
observation of the dog's behaviour and
physical condition allows for adjustments
to the supplementation plan as needed.

By addressing potential problems related
to health, behaviour, and anxiety, tissue
salts contribute to the overall well-being
and resilience of dogs during this critical
stage of development.

Thriving in 3rd Year to Seniority

Tissue Salts as Sustainers of Health in Dogs from their 3rd year to senior.

As dogs gracefully transition from their third year onward, they enter a phase that demands special attention to their changing health needs. Tissue salts, celebrated for their targeted cellular support, emerge as invaluable aids in promoting overall well-being and addressing the common challenges faced by dogs in their mature years. This section delves into how tissue salts can offer support during this stage, addressing potential problems, and issue's that dogs may experience as they journey towards their senior years. Head on over to our website for our dedicated digital course on how to use homeopathy in the Golden Years for your dog.

Understanding the Challenges of the Mature Years:

Dogs entering their third year and beyond often face a range of age-related issues, from joint stiffness to cognitive changes.

Tissue salts provide a natural and holistic approach to support their health during this significant life stage.

The bigger the dog the shorter its lifespan and where as some smaller breeds reach 15 plus years easily, some of our giant breeds struggle past 7 years old.

Common support issues in Dogs from the 3rd Year to Seniority:
Joint Stiffness and Arthritis:
Common Conerns may include reduced mobility, stiffness, and signs of arthritis.

Tissue Salt: Calcarea Fluorica (Calc Fluor) supports joint health, offering relief from stiffness and aiding in managing arthritis Issues.

Digestive Sensitivities:
Upset stomach, indigestion, or changes in appetite.

Tissue Salt: Natrum phosphoricum (Nat Phos) regulates pH balance, aiding in digestion and preventing acidosis, providing relief from digestive discomfort.

Dental Health Issues:

Dental problems, such as weakened teeth or gum issues.

Tissue Salt: Calcarea Fluorica (Calc Fluor) supports dental health, potentially contributing to stronger teeth and healthier gums.

Cognitive Decline:

Common Concern's may include memory loss, confusion, or changes in behaviour.

Tissue Salt: Kali phosphoricum (Kali Phos) supports mental alertness and may contribute to cognitive health in aging dogs.

Skin and Coat Issues:

Common concern's can include dry skin, dull coat, or skin irritations.

Tissue Salt: Silicea supports skin health and may contribute to a healthier coat.

Immune System Support:

Common issue's which show as an increased vulnerability to infections.

Tissue Salt: Ferrum phosphoricum (Ferr Phos) enhances oxygenation, supporting a robust immune response.

Incorporating Tissue Salts into Senior Dog Care:
By using tissue salts during a dog's mature years making use of regular observation of the dog's behaviour and physical condition will allow for adjustments to the supplementation plan as needed.

Tissue salts offer a gentle and natural approach to supporting dogs as they navigate the challenges of their mature years. By addressing common health concerns and promoting overall well-being, tissue salts contribute to a higher quality of life for dogs entering their seniority, allowing them to age gracefully and maintain vitality in their golden years.

Aging Gracefully

Tissue Salts as Nurturers of Well-being in Dogs during their Golden Years

The senior years of a dog's life bring forth unique challenges that require careful attention to their changing health needs. Tissue salts, esteemed for their targeted cellular support, become steadfast companions in promoting comfort, vitality, and overall well-being during this stage. This section explores how tissue salts can offer support for various issues commonly faced by senior dogs, including diminishing eyesight, hearing problems, incontinence, weight loss, mobility challenges, grumpiness, dental health, and general support for common issues associated with aging. As we all age the imbalance of these vital minerals diminish and by incorporating the tissue salts into our daily routines we can start to replenish our dwindling resources.

Understanding the Challenges of the Senior Years:

Senior dogs often experience a spectrum of age-related issues that can affect their physical health, cognitive function, and emotional well-being.

Tissue salts provide a natural and holistic approach to support them through these challenges.

Common support issues in Senior Dogs:

Diminishing Eyesight and Hearing Problems:
Common concerns may include reduced visual acuity, hearing loss, bumping into things or sensory decline.

Tissue Salt: Calcarea Phosphorica (Calc Phos) supports overall vitality, potentially contributing to the wellbeing of sensory organs.

Incontinence:
Common concerns may include: Difficulty controlling bladder function. Urinating whilst in their bed asleep.

Tissue Salt: Natrum muriaticum (Nat Mur) supports fluid balance and may aid in managing mild cases of incontinence.

Weight Loss:
Common issues may include Unintended weight loss despite a regular diet with no changes in food.

Tissue Salt: Natrum phosphoricum (Nat Phos) regulates pH balance, aiding in digestion and preventing acidosis, potentially supporting weight maintenance.

Mobility Problems:
Stiffness, Cracking joints and discomfort, or difficulty moving.

Tissue Salt: Calcarea Fluorica (Calc Fluor) supports joint health, offering relief from stiffness and aiding in managing mobility challenges.

Grumpiness:
Behavioural changes, irritability, or mood swings.

Tissue Salt: Kali phosphoricum (Kali Phos) may help alleviate stress and nervousness, promoting emotional balance and reducing grumpiness.

Dental Health Support:
Dental issues such as weakened teeth or gum problems. Reluctance to eat, dropping food on the floor.

Tissue Salt: Silicea supports dental health, potentially contributing to stronger teeth and healthier gums.

General Support for Common issues:
Various age-related issues such as immune vulnerability.

Tissue Salt: Ferrum phosphoricum (Ferr Phos) enhances oxygenation, supporting a robust immune response.

Incorporating Tissue Salts into Senior Dog Care:
It is vital as Pet guardians, to collaborate with vets and caregivers to design a targeted supplementation plan using tissue salts during a dog's senior years. Regular observation of the dog's behaviour and physical condition allows for adjustments to the supplementation plan as needed. Keeping a record of

weight and condition can be useful throughout a dog's life but will play a key part in their senior years to help senior dogs navigate the challenges associated with aging. Tissue salts contribute to a higher quality of life for dogs in their senior years, allowing them to age with grace and maintain comfort and vitality

Compassionate Care

Tissue Salts as Soothing Companions in a Dog's Final Journey

The final weeks or days of a dog's life bring about a period that demands utmost care, comfort, and compassion. Tissue salts, revered for their targeted cellular support, become invaluable allies in providing relief and support during this delicate stage. This section explores how tissue salts can offer comfort for common issues faced by dogs in their last weeks or days, addressing issues and supporting the to enhance their well-being as they approach the end of their journey.

Understanding the Challenges of the Final Stage:

In the twilight of a dog's life, various physical and emotional challenges may arise, requiring specialised attention to ensure a peaceful transition. Tissue salts provide a gentle and holistic approach to supporting dogs during this sensitive time.

Common support issues in Dogs in Their Final Weeks or Days:
Pain Management:
Discomfort, restlessness, or signs of pain.

Tissue Salt: Magnesia Phosphorica (Mag Phos) may aid in providing relief from muscle cramps and discomfort, promoting a more comfortable state.

Anxiety and Stress:
Common Issues may include: Behavioural changes, restlessness, or heightened anxiety.

Tissue Salt: Kali phosphoricum (Kali Phos) may help alleviate stress and nervousness, promoting a sense of calm and comfort.

Loss of Appetite:
Reduced interest in food or difficulty eating.

Tissue Salt: Natrum phosphoricum (Nat Phos) regulates pH balance, aiding in digestion and supporting appetite.

Immune Support:
Increased vulnerability to infections or illnesses.

Tissue Salt: Ferrum phosphoricum (Ferr Phos) enhances oxygenation, offering gentle support to the immune system.

Emotional Support:

Changes in behaviour, withdrawal, or signs of emotional distress.

Tissue Salt: Kali muriaticum (Kali Mur) supports emotional balance, providing gentle relief during times of emotional strain.

Incorporating Tissue Salts into End-of-Life Care:

During the last weeks or days, pet guardians, caregivers, and veterinarians can work together to create a supportive care plan that includes tissue salts. The specific tissue salts and their dosages can be adjusted based on the individual needs and issues of the dog.

Tissue salts offer a tender and compassionate approach to caring for dogs in their final weeks or days. By addressing common challenges associated with this stage of life, tissue salts can contribute to the comfort and well-being of the beloved canine companion, providing solace to both the pet and its caregivers during this poignant and inevitable part of the life journey.

If possible then a home visit for that final time may be discussed with your vet as that time approaches. Keeping the dog comfortable and in familiar surroundings with their guardians close by.

Quick guide to the tissue salts.

1. **Calc Fluor:** Loss of elasticity, calcification of the joints.
2. **Calc Phos:** Weakness in muscle, bones and teeth.
3. **Calc Sulph:** Antiseptic for removing pus.
4. **Ferr Phos:** Poor circulation, frequent infections.
5. **Kali Murr:** Lymphatic and glandular detox.
6. **Kali Phos:** Nerve issues.
7. **Kali Sulph:** Skin disorders and hormone imbalances.
8. **Mag Phos:** Muscular cramps and nerve spasms.
9. **Nat Mur:** The water balancer, Dryness, oedemas.
10. **Nat Phos:** Acidity, stiff muscles and joint swelling.
11. **Nat Sulph:** Excessive bile and high level of toxicity within the body.
12. **Silica:** Weakness in Skin, Hair, nails.

Quick reference Chart tissue salts.

Condition	Main Tissue Salt	Secondary Tissue Salt
Abrasions'	Ferrum Phos	Kali Phos
Abscess	Silica	Calc Sulph
Acidity	Nat Sulph	Nat Phos
Allergies (Digestive)	Nat Sulph	Nat Phos
Allergies (Respiratory)	Nat Mur	Kali Mur
Allergies (Skin)	Kali Sulph	Nat Mur
Anaemia	Calc Phos	Ferrum Phos
Anxiety	Kali Phos	Calc Phos
Appetite (Poor)	Calc Phos	Silica
Arthritis	Nat Phos	Ferrum Phos
Bones (Weak)	Calc Phos	Silica
Colic	Mag Phos	Nat Sulph
Constipation	Dry Nat Mur	Mucous Kali Mur
Cramps	Muscle Mag Phos	Digestive Calc Phos
Dermatitis	Kali Sulph	Nat Mur
Detox – Blood	Calc Sulph	Kali Sulph
Detox Skin	Kali Sulph	Kali Mur
Diarrhoea	Nat Phos	Nat Sulph
Epitasis- Nose bleed	Ferr Phos	Calc Phos
Fear	Kali Phos	Silica

Condition	Main Tissue Salt	Secondary Tissue Salt
Flatulence	Nat Sulph	Nat Phos
Gas Belching	Nat Phos	Calc Phos
Growing Pains	Calc Phos	Ferrum Phos
Hormonal Imbalance	Kali Sulph	Calc Phos
Immunity (Poor)	Calc Phos	Kali Phos
Indigestion	Nat Sulph	Nat Phos
Inflammation	Ferr Phos	Nat Mur
Joint Pain	Nat Phos	Ferrum Phos
Kidney Stones	Nat Phos	Nat Sulph
Nails (Brittle)	Silica	Calc Fluor
Osteoarthritis	Calc Fluor	Nat Mur
Rheumatism	Nat Phos	Nat Sulph
Ringworm	Kali Sulph	Kali Mur
Skin Disorders	Kali Phos	Nat Mur
Sores (Slow to Heal)	Calc Sulph	Kali Phos
Spasms	Mag Phos	Calc Fluor
Sprains (Muscular)	Ferrum Phos	Kali Phos
Stress	Mag Phos	Nat Phos
Swelling	Nat Sulph	Nat Mur
Teething	Calc Phos	Calc Fluor
Travel Sickness	Nat Sulph	Kali Phos
Vomiting	Nat Sulph	Nat Phos

Areas of the body and indicated tissue salts.

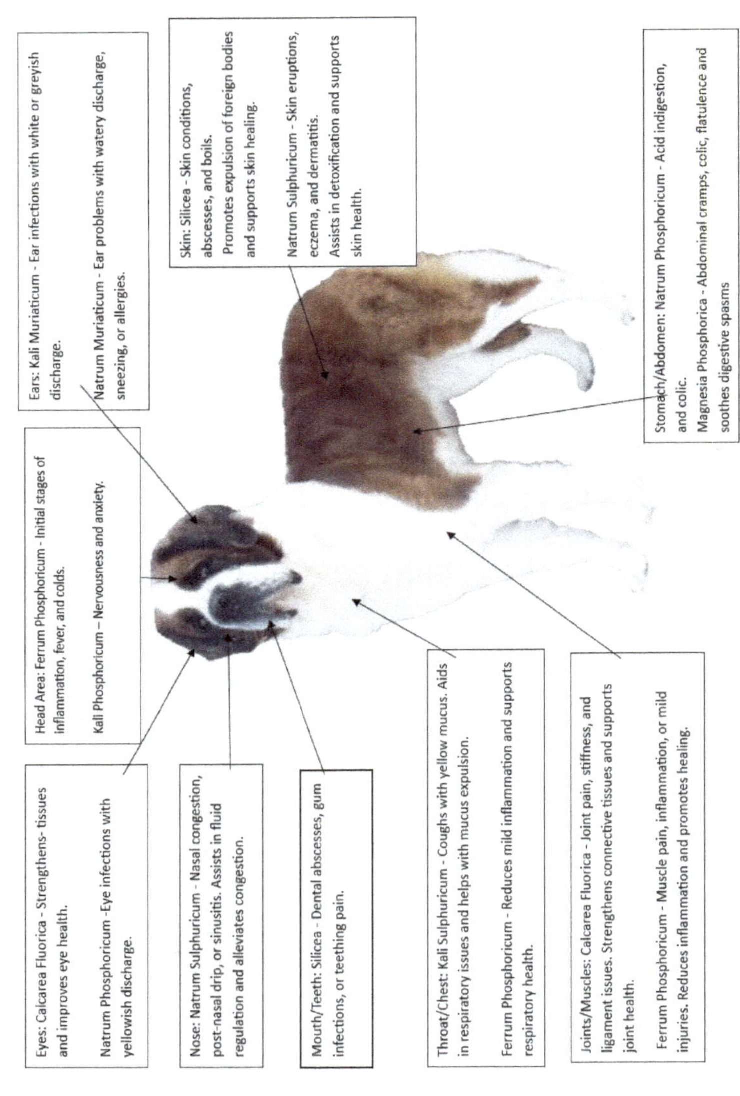

Index

This index provides a comprehensive guide to the Health Conditions Supported by the 12 biochemic tissue salts in canine care, making it easy to find the appropriate remedy for various conditions.

Coming soon

THE ESSENTIAL GUIDE FOR TISSUE SALTS FOR CATS.

THE ESSENTIAL GUIDE FOR TISSUE SALTS FOR HORSES.

THE ESSENTIAL GUIDE FOR TISSUE SALTS ON THE FARM

Coaching Sessions available on our website

www.homeopathypetcoaching.com

Digital courses and informative blogs available on

www.homeopathypetcoaching.com

How to use the Helios Pet Kit